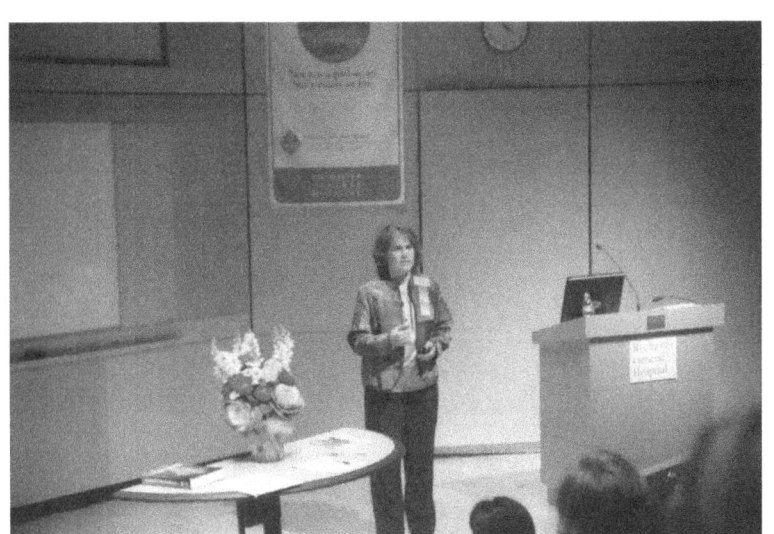

Jean Oswald, R.N., CCA, Aromatherapist

Contents

Introduction to Jean Oswald, RN, CCA

This is Robert Rodgers from <u>Parkinsons Recovery</u>. It is exciting for me to have an interview with Jean Oswald who has been working as a registered nurse in <u>Rochester, New York</u> for 14 years; she is a Certified Clinical <u>Aromatherapist</u> and has been using essential oils now for 10 years. This is something I wanted everyone with the symptoms of Parkinson's to know more about since essential oils have the potential to provide significant relief for their symptoms.

When I use the term "essential oils" what is that exactly? What is an essential oil?

True 'essential oils' refer to a pure, therapeutic grade essential oil. Essential oils are actually the liquid extract, the " life blood" of plants, trees, shrubs, flowers and plants.   They come from organically grown plants harvested at the peak of season when they have ideal levels of therapeutic compounds inside. These plants undergo <u>steam distillation</u> over low temperatures and low pressure lasting a long period of time. They are very different from "perfume grade" oils that can be purchased at local health food stores or retail stores like "Bath & Body Works." The therapeutic grade oils I am referring to are actually nature's medicine right from the earth.

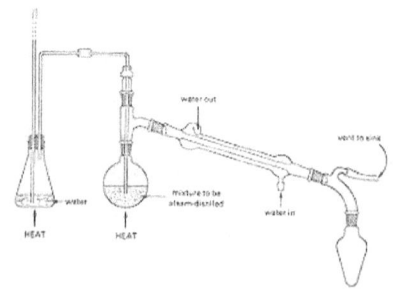

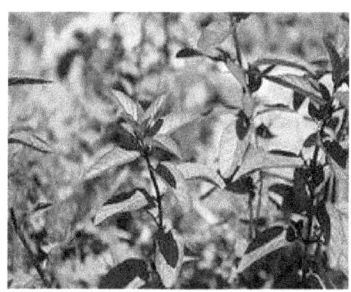 *They are more potent than the plant forms of <u>Peppermint</u>[1] or <u>Basil</u> that you grow in your garden as well. I say this because, when*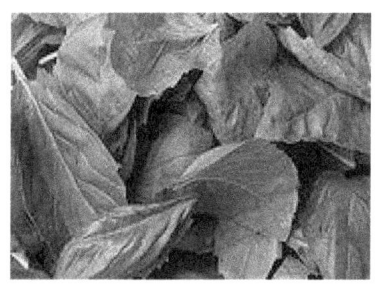

you pick the peppermint or basil from your garden, its life force will measure at a lower 'frequency' or 'vibration' over time as it dries.

*Essential oils will measure at a higher MHz, with more of their life force*Error! Bookmark not defined. *intact. Essential oils are a concentrated form of the plant. Some essential oils require hundreds of pounds of plant material to make a single ounce of essential oil. So the end result will be far more potent than dried herbs. Essential oils also smell wonderful and they have many medicinal properties.*

If I were interested in getting some essential oils to help with my symptoms such as tremors and rigidity, would I first purchase a 12 ounce bottle at a health food store and put them on my skin as I might put any lotion on my body?

---

[1] *Peppermint (Mentha piperita) has a strong, clean, fresh, minty aroma. One of the oldest and most highly regarded herbs for soothing digestion, it may also restore digestive efficiency.* Jean Valnet MD studied peppermint's supportive effect on the liver and respiratory systems. Other scientists have also researched peppermint's role in improving taste and smell when inhaled. Dr. William N. Dember of the University of Cincinnati studied peppermint's ability to improve concentration and mental sharpness. Alan Hirsch MD studied peppermint's ability to directly affect the brain's satiety center, which triggers a sensation of fullness after meals. This powerful essential oil is often diluted before topical application. Peppermint may also be used to enhance the flavor of food and water. Peppermint has an approximate ORAC of 373,455 (TE/L). TE/L is expressed as micromole Trolox equivalent per liter.*

If you did that, you might not have the response you are hoping for. Most people do not know about the importance of using a therapeutic grade underline essential oil. So, they will do just what you suggested.

But let me give you an example of what could happen. Let's say you love the smell of Lavender[2]. You go into your local natural health food store. You see lavender on the shelf and notice it only costs $6, so you buy it and bring it home. You put it your kitchen window sill.

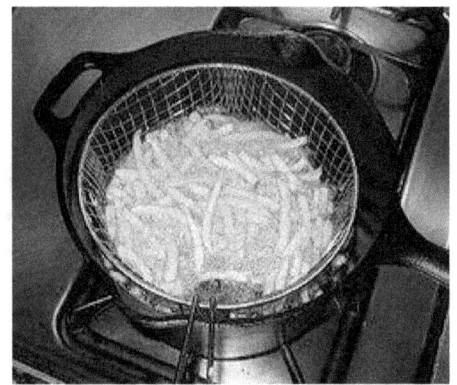

A week later you are cooking. You burn yourself using the fry pan. You may remember that Lavender is frequently helpful for burns so you reach for that bottle. That bottle of lavender could actually contain more lavendin than lavandula angustifolia. Lavendin contains camphor which can actually turn a second degree burn into a third degree burn! Yikes!

---

[2] *Lavandula angustifolia) has a fresh, sweet, floral, herbaceous aroma that is soothing and refreshing. Because it is the most versatile of all essential oils, no home should be without it. Lavender is an adaptogen, and therefore can assist the body when adapting to stress or imbalances. It is a great aid for relaxing and winding down before bedtime, yet has balancing properties that can also boost stamina and energy. Therapeutic-grade lavender is highly regarded for skin and beauty. It may be used to soothe and cleanse common cuts, bruises, and skin irritations. The French scientist René Gattefossé was among the first to discover these properties when he was severely burned in a laboratory explosion. Lavender may also be used to enhance the flavor of foods. Lavender has an approximate ORAC of 3,669 (TE/L). TE/L is expressed as micromole Trolox equivalent per liter.*

On the other hand <u>Lavandula angustifolia</u> would begin healing the skin very quickly. I have burned myself in the kitchen and can attest to this; in fact by using <u>lavandula angustifolia</u> I found that I don't even have a scar!

So I would say no, it is not a good idea to go into a natural food store and buy an essential oil that reads "pure, therapeutic grade." You see, today there are no standards in America for selling essential oils, so all a manufacturer is required to do is put one drop of pure essential oil in a bottle and then a label can be put on the bottle that says the entire bottle is pure, therapeutic grade. This is unfortunate but true. You really need to know the company you buy from!

In Europe (especially in France) physicians have been prescribing essential oils for decades. They have relationships with their distillers. They know they are getting a therapeutic grade essential oil. Pure essential oils are not extracted with solvents or toxic chemicals that can cause adverse reactions.

Therapeutic grade essential oils are distilled at low pressure and low temperature over long periods. These specific oils will be tested in a laboratory with an instrument called a gas chromatograph and mass spectrometer. This equipment shows which healing compounds are in the oils and the actual percentages of those specific compounds. In contrast, over- the- counter oils are considered 'perfume grade'.

I hope you can see that your source of essential oils is important.

How would I know what type of essential oil will help me? For example, if my symptoms are tremors and rigidity, are there specific essential oils that can help offer me some relief from my symptoms?

Yes there are specific oils that offer relief.

As an <u>aroma therapist</u> I can offer suggestions or you could work with a physician who understands <u>essential oils</u>. Usually people cannot get education on every topic so they go to a specialist. I do consultations for example. Many aroma therapists around the country also offer essential oil consultations.

You live in Rochester, New York. If I lived in California would I be able to get a consultation with you?

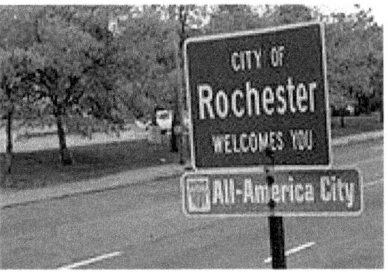

Sure. I do phone consultations.

So, in a consultation, we would talk about the issues that are problematic for the client and you would be able to sort through recommendations for what essential oils might help?

Yes. I am a <u>registered nurse</u>. Although I was trained in western medicine (which looks for a drug to treat a symptom), I prefer to understand the root cause of a disease and aim for healing those issues. Still, I will suggest an oil to help a symptom as we strive to make changes to bring the body back to balance.

You are an <u>aroma therapist</u>. Let's say I did a consultation with you. You recommended certain essential oils that I need. I then acquire these oils from you or from some source. How does aroma therapy work? Do I smell it or do I put it on my body?

There are actually many ways to use oils. Yes, you can smell them. That is one way. Fragrance travels through the olfactory system and goes directly to the limbic region of the brain where the <u>amygdala</u>

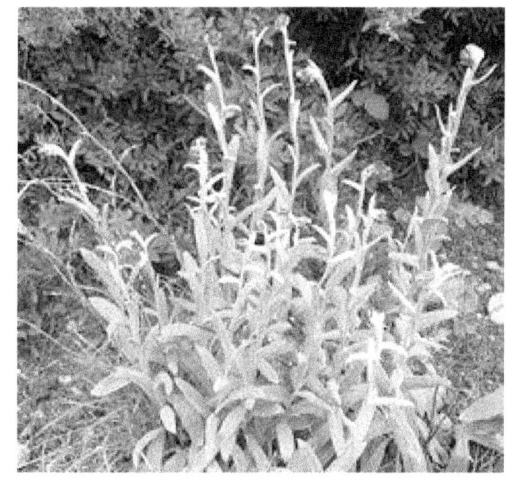

us resides. *Here emotions like anxiety and frustration can be released. Fragrance affects very much!*

You can also put essential oils on your body, on the skin. The tiny molecules are easily absorbed through every layer of the skin, sweat glands and nerves and can be detected in the bloodstream within minutes. This means they will circulate throughout the body very quickly to bring healing.

We can also take them internally in capsules or teaspoons of honey. Taking oils internally can provide a more therapeutic reaction, but it needs to be done under supervision of a professional who knows what they're talking about.

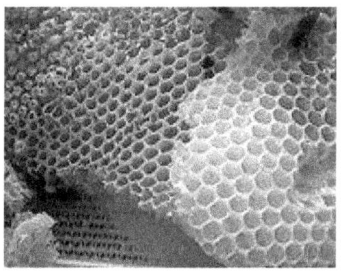

I'd like to back up a minute and say that there are different schools of thought on how to use essential oils:

- *The Germans recommend using essential oils via inhalation only.*

- *The French recommend inhalation, ingestion and <u>topical</u> use.*

- *The British prescribe diluting oils and using them primarily in massage.*

Actually, we can benefit most by using all of these methods.

So if we take the example of muscle rigidity in people with Parkinson's, aroma therapy massage could be very beneficial. Shirley Price is an aroma therapist who has written books for health care professionals. Her study called The Parkinson's Project was published online in "Positive Health" magazine. Her work found that aroma therapy massage was very beneficial in easing pain, rigidity and movement in general.

It sounds like there are a lot of options. You can actually ingest them? You can put them in liquids?

Essential oils are the end product of distillation, so they come in liquid form. They are the liquid extract from plants, remember? I take essential oils in capsule myself when I am feeling run down or if I am around people who have colds and sore throats. I did it this week and knocked a sore throat out of my system within 24 hours.

Are they sold in big bottles that would be, for example, 10 ounces or are they smaller bottles with only a few ounces?

I buy essential oils online from a company called Young Living. They are the largest manufacturer of essential oils in the United States. In business for 13 years, this company has stringent benchmarks for distilling and selling therapeutic grade oils. I have been to their distillery in Utah and I have personally met Gary Young who is the CEO.

I would describe him as having an Indiana Jones personality because he has done the legwork himself in building his company from the ground up. He has studied with experts around the world to really understand what it takes to make good quality oils…… from growing the seeds all the way to packaging it and sending it to you. Gary is committed to healing on a cellular level because of his own personal story. I think you can read it online……

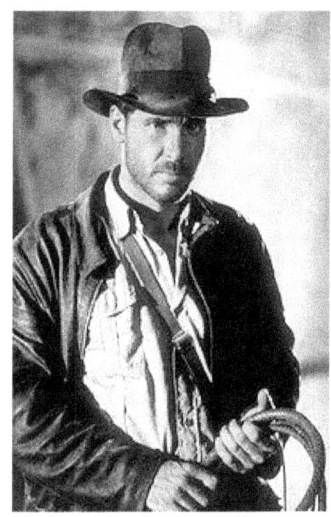

Young Living's oils come in very small bottles. The biggest bottle I have is actually 15

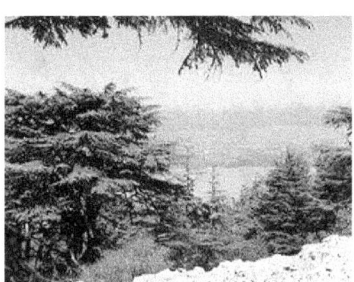

milliliters. That is half an ounce. They are small but at the same time these bottles have up to 300 drops in them. They are very concentrated. You will only need a couple of drops in an application, so the bottle of oil can last you two to three months. When people first hear how much they cost, they sound expensive. But, like I said, you only need a little bit.

There is a big variation in the cost of the oils. That really depends on where it comes from around the world. High quality Frankincense is scarce right now as is Helichrysum[3] .

When companies approach Gary to sell their oils to him, he is careful to look at the GC/MS breakdown of compounds in the oil. He knows what percentage of specific compounds he is looking for because he knows what properties those compounds offer us in healing ability. This means that he won't accept a batch that falls below his standard even when he is criticized for this.

---

[3] *Helichrysum (Helichrysum italicum) is known for its restorative properties and provides excellent support to the skin, liver, and nervous system.* Scoring an amazing 17,430 on the ORAC scale, Helichrysum also provides a defense against harmful free radicals, making it a vital ingredient in several Young Living blends.*

Let's say I had a consultation with you. You recommend certain oils. I receive them in the mail and I start to apply them. I find that one of the oils in particular gives me wonderful relief. I am a pretty intensive person, so I start putting a lot of that particular oil on my skin. Can I overdo it? Can I put too much oil on myself?

Yes, you can. And you can waste a lot of oil too. There are few fatal toxicity cases that occur, but they are almost always dose related. I keep Robert Tisserand's book on my desk: Essential Oil Safety: A Guide for Healthcare Professionals so that I can look up information as I need to.

Also, it helps that these bottles come with drop dispensers. They only pour a drop at a time. Even for children it would take a whole 15 milliliter bottle to hurt a child. Because of the drop's dispenser they are much safer to use.

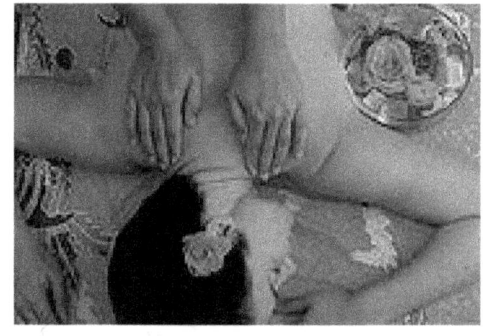

Besides the safety issue, there wouldn't be a need to use 10 or more drops on the skin. Remember I said that they are more potent than herbs because they are concentrated? They are powerful in small amounts. I offer a special treatment in my office called Raindrop Technique but I only use about 6 drops at a time for this unique treatment. If I were instructing someone to use these oils at home, I would be telling them to use 2 or 3 drops at the most.

The raindrop treatment is like a <u>massage</u>?

No, Raindrop Technique is not a massage. It was developed by Gary Young about 15-20 years ago and it is based on his research with essential oils as antimicrobial agents, his knowledge of VitaFlex technique and its reflex points on the feet and information on finger stroking that he learned when he lived with the Lakota people in South Dakota. This technique has a powerful effect on the muscles and nervous system.

I have also been reading about a protocol that Gary has been using at his clinic in Ecuador for the past couple of years. It is called the neuroauricular technique (pronounced 'noricular') and it is performed with essential oils and a glass probe (lightly touching the skin) at the top of the brain stem and down the spine.

There is a lot of interest in this technique specifically for people with Parkinson's disease because there seems to be a correlation between stimulating that part of the brain stem (the top where endorphins, neurotransmitters, enzymes, and hormones either get congested there or don't move easily down the brain stem) and the improvement of connections between the nervous system and the muscles.

Has there been research to evaluate the impact of essential oils?

Yes. There are thousands of articles online and in journals about ways that essential oils can help with common problems like mood, chronic pain, digestive issues, sleep and more. For example, I subscribe to an international online data base in France. It helps me identify studies done on certain essential oils that I can share with my clients.

I recently accessed 3 studies describing how limonene helped prevent breast, liver and lung cancer. I have a folder full of clinical studies on specific physical issues where essential oils have been shown to be helpful. I also have stories from individuals who have found some improvement with Parkinson's symptoms from using essential oils, but you need to understand that Parkinson's disease doesn't go away with one essential oil application.

In America, the primary clinical studies that are done are funded by pharmaceutical companies. Pharmaceutical companies cannot make any money on natural plants. You cannot put a patent on something like peppermint, Basil or Cedarwood Pharmaceutical companies are not interested in funding these studies. There are therefore few studies that examine the effect of essential oils using human subjects.

There are different organizations across the world that are starting to come together, even the National Institute of Health. If you go on www.pubmed.gov you will see 7,000 postings[4] of studies that have been done with essential oils.. Even though I have been in the audience where doctors are talking about essential oils, this work is still considered 'new' to most doctors.

What if an individual has problems with muscle rigidity and it is very difficult for them to move with ease. What is an essential oil that might help relieve that particular symptom?

There are a few essential oils that can be helpful. But because each person's body chemistry is different, you might need to try a few before you find the right one. This requires some patience.

---

[4] *Click on the pubmet.gov link and type in the search window the term "essential oils" and at least 7,835 entries (as of November, 2008) will be found.*

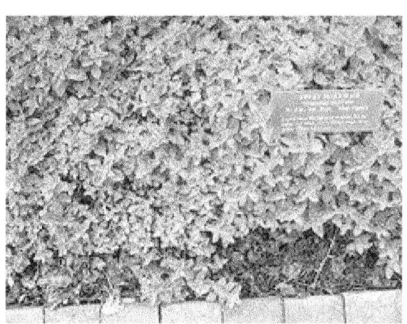

Gary Young's <u>*Essential Oils Integrative Medical Guide*</u> *suggests using* <u>*Juniper*</u>*,* <u>*Peppermint*</u> *and* <u>*Vitex*</u> *essential oils. I would suggest applying a drop or two of these oils right on specific muscles that feel tight. Muscle rigidity might lessen with the help of* <u>*Marjoram*</u> *essential oil.*

Using these oils in a massage or putting them directly on the skin along the spine (as we do in Raindrop Technique) can be helpful. When we use a blend of essential oils, there is a synergy that occurs where many gentle, but subtle effects can make a difference for the person.

How about the problem of tremors? What essential oils might be recommended to relieve that symptom?

<u>*Basil*</u> *is the first oil that comes to mind or* <u>*Frankincense*</u>*, because they are well known for their anti-spasmodic action.*

A problem some people have is with excessive salivation. Are there any essential oils that come to mind specifically for that symptom?

I would have to do some research on what causes the salivation to understand what would support that best.

This is a weird one - how about <u>insomnia</u>?

That one is not so surprising. Taking a look at the common drugs on the market, you can see a lot of people suffer from insomnia. There are many causes of insomnia as well, so there are many options in essential oils: <u>*Lavender*</u> *comes to mind of course, but so does* <u>*Roman Chamomile*</u> *and* <u>*Valerian*</u>*.*

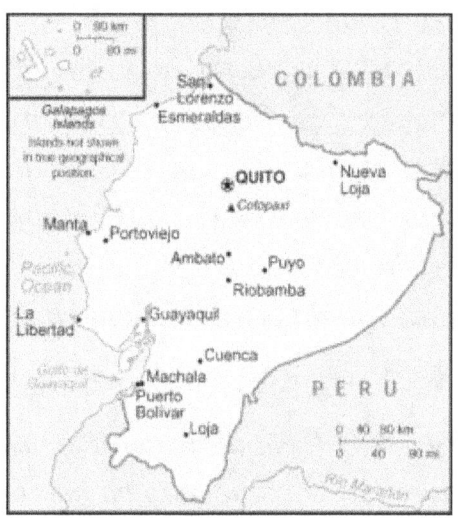

There is a new essential oil blend that Young Living made last year combining Ruta, from the rainforest in Equador, with Valerian and Lavender and they call it RutaVaLa[5]. This oil has helped me fall asleep better than any other and I sleep soundly! Sometimes I use that Citrus Blend called Peace & Calming or the Lavender for a long time and find that I need to make a switch. I have a variety of oils to choose from.

Many people I interview talk quite extensively about stress and how that affects them. When they are under extreme stress their symptoms flare up. Can essential oils address the problems that stress creates?

I think that's a loaded question really because in America we tend to live in what I will call "sympathetic overdrive" If you have visited other parts of the world you can see that other cultures live a more "laid back" existence. Here we move quickly, have long lists of things to do, want everything 'instantly' and this keeps our bodies in the 'fight or flight' mode. That 'lifestyle' is a dangerous precursor to disease. In other words, we create much of our own stress.

I encourage every client to lie down in 'corpse pose' for 15 minutes/day or 15 minutes/day 3-4 times a week. This alone can make a difference. Can essential oils help with stress?

---

[5] *RutaVaLa promotes relaxation of the body and mind. It helps ease tension and relieve stress. The blend helps overcome negative feelings while encouraging a positive attitude and comfort.*

Definitely. One of the best things to do is put a drop of essential oil into the palm of your hand and rub your hands together. Then hold your hands over your mouth and nose, close your eyes and inhale. The fragrance alone can make a difference.

Balsam Fir[6] is a useful oil for almost any of the symptoms we have already covered. Balsam Fir really helps the body relax. It is a good anti-inflammatory essential oil. For stress, that is the first one I think of. But again, Frankincense, Lavender and Cedarwood are very good for that as well.

You give talks to many different audiences about essential oils – to health care communities, doctors, nurses, physical therapists and other interested groups. Are you still available to give talks to groups?

I love sharing the information about essential oils. Last fall I gave a talk at one of our local hospitals on two clinical studies that have been done… One of them was done in a laboratory; the other in a nursing home in New Jersey. The studies found that essential oils are effective in killing superbugs like MRSA.

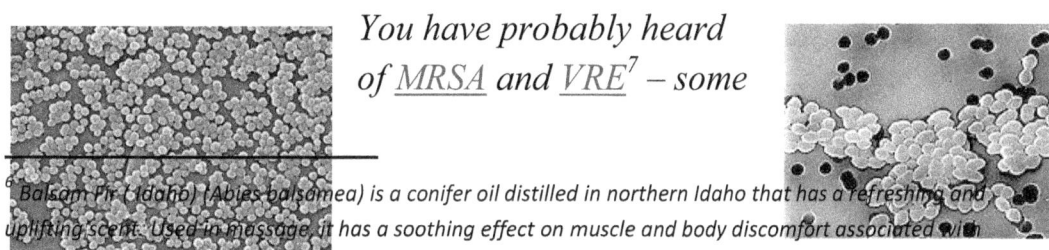

You have probably heard of MRSA and VRE[7] – some

---

[6] *Balsam Fir (Idaho) (Abies balsamea) is a conifer oil distilled in northern Idaho that has a refreshing and uplifting scent. Used in massage, it has a soothing effect on muscle and body discomfort associated with exercise*

[7] *Vancomycin-resistant enterococcus (VRE)*

of those really strong bugs that the big gun <u>antibiotics</u> *can't seem to help? Essential oils have been tested both in the lab and in clinical settings and found to be effective in destroying airborne bacteria.*

For me, going into a hospital and having doctors and nurses tell me how this is good news feels wonderful. It is helping to change the face of medicine.

There are some reports that pathogens and bacterial infections confound the symptoms of Parkinson's. It sounds like essential oils have the potential to address those pathogens?

Yes, very much so. And that is why essential oils are so special because there is a synergy amongst the molecules within a single essential oil. If you consider the fact that there are hundreds of molecules in one single essential oil, then you begin to understand the scope of how an essential oil can confuse the microbes. Penicillin always looks the same as a chemical compound, but essential oils have too many compounds for a microbe to figure out how to get through the cell wall. They will be more effective at killing microbes!

Obviously people who live in states other than <u>New York</u> and in other countries will have difficulty getting you to come and give talks. Are you available to give conference calls to Parkinson's support groups?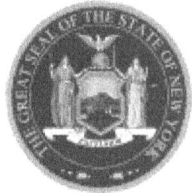

Definitely. If you want to fly me out to Washington state or Albuquerque, New Mexico (or wherever) I would be delighted to come and talk.

If a person would like to have a specific consultation with you about symptoms they are experiencing, how do they go about doing that?

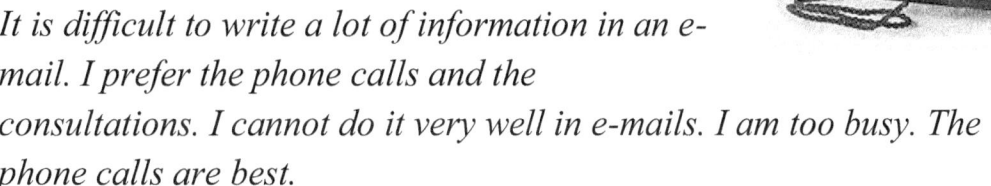

My phone number in the United States is 1-585-872-6242. My e-mail address is: jean@compassionateconsulting.net. And my website is www.compassionateconsulting.net

It is difficult to write a lot of information in an e-mail. I prefer the phone calls and the consultations. I cannot do it very well in e-mails. I am too busy. The phone calls are best.

Your career has been fascinating Jean. I know you have been very intensively involved in the medical establishment as a nurse and have worked in some very intensive care medical environments. What encouraged you to make this shift and work more in a field many people do not know much about – the area of essential oils and aroma therapy?

After several years of working in a local hospital I wanted to help people in a more personal way. "High tech" nursing can save lives, but it also felt impersonal. I also believe we need to help people understand what causes illness so that we can heal from the inside out.

I was fortunate to meet a nurse about five years ago who introduced me to a doctor who chaired the integrative health committee in our local medical society. We have about 1,700 physicians in the medical society. They had asked about a dozen years ago to develop this integrative health committee because so many of their patients were asking doctors:

"Do you know about acupuncture?"

"Can I go see a chiropractor? The pain in my back isn't getting better."

"What do you think about herbs? Will they interact with my drugs? Are they safe?"

I was so excited to join this group because for years in the hospital setting and in the community home health care setting I was feeling western medicine was incomplete.

I am a sensitive soul myself. I react strongly to drugs. I do much better with natural medicine. And as a mother I wanted something better than a prescription.

I have five children and I have been using essential oils with my kids for years. They have gone on to college with their own set of oils. They love to call home and tell me how they are working for them and how they are sharing them with friends.

I was very excited being a part of the Integrative Health Committee and being supported by local practitioners. Everybody from <u>Reiki</u> masters to <u>massage</u> therapists to <u>chiropractors</u> to pediatric integrative health doctors…. It inspired me to begin doing what I love. I had been using the oils for such a long time, so I had a powerful tool to help people on an individual basis.

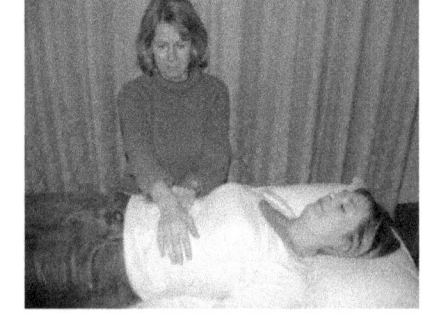

I feel that there is so much more that is needed than drugs and surgery. Primarily that is what doctors learn in medical school. I think we all know it is incomplete and sometimes not the right answer for people.

So, that is how I really got into this – through the encouragement of one of the doctors on this committee to share information about essential oils with people. This is what I have been doing and I absolutely love it.

This is not a sideline for you. You are not doing this part time. This is a full time commitment for you. Is this right?

It is definitely a full time commitment to me; in fact I need to find more balance in my life. I get so passionate about sharing the oils that I forget to eat or stop and go for a walk in the sunshine.

You are not doing the intensive care nursing work anymore?

I am weaning away from traditional nursing jobs. I work two days a week in an infusion center and devote 3-4 days/week to my own business.

What is so marvelous about essential oils is that it is a noninvasive therapy. You are not cutting into anybody. It is a very gentle but powerful therapy.

The oils also amplify any energy work. There are all sorts of ways essential oils amplify the work of Reiki, craniosacral or Emotional Freedom Technique that you might already be doing.

If you understand vibration and frequency of living things the essential oils that are pure, therapeutic grade actually raise the vibration. That is another way that they help us.

That will be of interest to many people who are reading and listening to this. Many people are getting craniosacral work or Bowen therapy or some type of energy work now. It will be interesting for them to explore the possibility of supplementing that work with some of these essential oils.

That is exciting.

> **You mention that you do consultations with people. It is one thing to say you do these, but it is quite another to get a sense of how this works. Are you available to be a guest on another teleseminar? I could invite several people to join us. You could basically do a live consultation with them while others listen. Would you be willing to do that?**

That would be wonderful. I would need to ask them to complete an intake form before the consultation. Background information is very important so I can feel the broader scope of what someone is dealing with.

We will do that. People can then get a real sense of what an essential oils consultation is all about.

Thank you for being available to talk about this wonderful, new, powerful area of aroma therapy and essential oils that many people with the symptoms of Parkinson's know very little about.

Index

www.ingramcontent.com/pod-product-compliance
Lightning Source LLC
Chambersburg PA
CBHW052043280526
45791CB00010B/3066